AF427079

Type 2 Diabetes

How to Eat Better, Lower Blood Sugar, and Manage Diabetes

Christina Neal

Table of Contents

CHAPTER ONE

An Overview of Type 2 Diabetes

According to the American Diabetes Association, diabetes currently ranks as the No. 7 leading cause of death in the United States, affecting more than 29 million people, or 9.3% of the population. The costs of medicine and hospitalization, and other health costs related to this "silent killer" are more than $245 billion in the United States alone.

What Is Diabetes?

Diabetes is a common and prevalent disease that occurs when the blood glucose levels in your blood get too high. In general, blood glucose comes from the food you eat and is the main source of energy for your body to perform routine and necessary tasks. Most of the food that you eat is broken down into glucose by the body and this glucose is sent through your blood to every part of your body for energy.

Many hormones play an important role in converting the food you eat into glucose. One such hormone is called insulin and this is made by the organ called pancreas. The insulin hormone is responsible for taking the glucose from your blood stream and delivering them to each individual cell.

Diabetics either do not produce enough insulin due to a malfunctioning pancreas (type 1), or their body's cells do not adequately respond to the insulin circulating through their bloodstream (type 2). As a result, the person's blood is flooded with glucose.

Symptoms of Diabetes

Symptoms of diabetes will vary depending on the type, as well as any other health problems the person may be experiencing. However, most diabetics experience one or more of the following:

Frequent Urination and Unusual Thirst
One of the primary and most noticeable symptoms of diabetes is frequent urination. This particular symptom commonly manifests at night, and those suffering from the condition usually find themselves arising from bed 2-4 times each night for the purpose of emptying a full bladder. Frequent urination is almost always accompanied by excessive thirst. This symptom is very common with all types of diabetes.

Extreme Hunger
A sudden increase in appetite is also one of the symptoms of diabetes. This particular symptom is much more common with juvenile diabetes than gestational or type 2 diabetes. In many cases, such hunger is accompanied by the urge to binge on carbohydrates and starchy foods.

Unusual Weight Loss
Unexplained weight loss is often seen in the early stages of diabetes. While weight loss is a normal result of calorie restriction and exercise, it should never occur for no reason. Unexplained weight loss may be a symptom of all three types of diabetes.

Extreme Fatigue and Irritability
Irritability and fatigue often accompany abnormally high blood sugar. A person may also experience listlessness, sleepiness, aggressive mood swings or a feeling of stupor, all of which are most common in juveniles suffering from the disorder.

Frequent Infections

Along with all the aforementioned symptoms, frequent infections, especially yeast infections, can be a hallmark sign of the presence of diabetes. In addition, infections or cuts that are slow to heal are sometimes a symptom of the disorder, as the decreased circulation that accompanies the condition often slows the healing process. These symptoms are more often seen with type 2 diabetes.

Blurred Vision

Symptoms of adult onset or gestational diabetes sometimes include vision changes, most often in the form of blurred vision, as high blood sugar causes the lens of the eye to swell. Many times, people are tempted to ignore such symptoms and assume they are the vision changes one experiences with age or an indication that new glasses are needed. Although this symptom can occur in juveniles, it is much more common in diabetics over age forty-five.

Tingling and Numbness in the Feet and Hands

The symptoms of all types of diabetes can include a numbness or a tingling sensation in the extremities. This is another complication associated with the aforementioned decrease in circulation caused by high glucose levels. However, tingling and numbness are also associated with other diseases and conditions, and therefore a medical doctor should be consulted in order to make a definitive diagnosis.

Type 2 Diabetes

Type 2 (adult onset) diabetes accounts for 90 percent of all cases and typically strikes after age 45. With this type of the disorder, the body's cells do not properly respond to the insulin that is present in the bloodstream, resulting in high glucose levels despite the fact that adequate insulin is being produced. Although type 2 diabetes is typically diagnosed after age 45, an increasing number of individuals under the age of 30 are being diagnosed with the disorder each year. Some of the known factors that can lead to type 2 diabetes are:

Lifestyle

Overweight and physical inactivity are two of the major causes of type 2 diabetes. When you carry a lot of body weight, it impacts the production of insulin and the amount that is available may not be enough to pass the glucose to every cell in your body. This leads to accumulation of glucose in the blood, thereby leading to diabetes.

Resistance to insulin

In some people, for unknown reasons, the muscle, liver, and fat cells do not use insulin well. This means, the pancreas is forced to produce more insulin as whatever it is producing currently may not be enough. Although the pancreas adapts to producing more, the inefficient usage of insulin by the other organs, makes it difficult to bridge the gap.

Genetic factors

Some races are more prone to diabetes due to genetic factors and the food that they have been eating for generations. For example, Southeast Asians who thrive on carbohydrate rich rice as their staple are more predisposed to diabetes.

Family history

A family history greatly increases your chances to get diabetes.

Hormonal diseases

Some hormonal diseases like Cushing's syndrome and hyperthyroidism may cause diabetes. In Cushing's syndrome, the body produces too much cortisol, a hormone known to induce stress and reduce the production of insulin. Likewise, in hyperthyroidism, the thyroid produces too much thyroid hormone that impacts insulin.

Diagnosis

To diagnose the disorder, most physicians first order a fasting glucose test. The test is relatively simple: blood is drawn after the patient has refrained from drinking or eating for at least eight hours, and the amount of glucose in his or her blood is measured. Readings of 100 milligrams per deciliter (mg/dL) or greater may indicate a problem. The findings are typically verified through a second and third test, and if subsequent readings are 100 or higher, the person will likely be diagnosed with high blood sugar.

The hemoglobin A1c test, also called A1C, HbA1c or glycated hemoglobin test, is another blood test used to measure blood glucose. This test measures the amount of glucose that is attached to the hemoglobin protein, and is reported as a percentage. The normal levels of hemoglobin A1c are between 4 to 5.6 percent. Diabetes is diagnosed when the A1c readings are equal to or higher than 6.5 percent.

CHAPTER TWO

Diabetes Complications

Although diabetes can be effectively managed, diabetes complications are always a possibility, and can ultimately lead to additional health problems. Below are some of the common complications experienced by diabetics:

Diabetic Neuropathy

Neuropathy is a condition that results from nerve damage due to the poor circulation that almost always accompanies diabetes. As time goes on, diabetics often develop this condition in various areas throughout their body. Although a person may have no symptoms, in most cases neuropathy causes pain, tingling and numbness in the hands, arms, legs and feet. Diabetic neuropathy is usually treated with physical therapy and medication, but maintaining an ideal weight may help to prevent it from developing.

Foot Problems

It is not uncommon for diabetics to develop foot problems. Due to neuropathy and overall poor circulation, many diabetics lose sensation in the soles of their feet or experience pain in this area. The best way to prevent these conditions from developing is to wear diabetic socks or anti-thrombotic stockings, both of which significantly increase circulation in the extremities.

An appropriate diabetic foot care regimen also includes daily foot washing with warm water and soap. Because many diabetics are insensitive to heat, care must be taken to test the water temperature before immersing one's feet. It is also wise for diabetics to inspect their feet on a daily basis: due to insensitivity, it is possible for a person to step on a sharp object or not feel something in his or her shoe, which can lead to long-term foot damage or other serious conditions such as toxic shock.

Moisturizing the skin of one's feet after bathing is vital. This is because the feet of diabetics no longer emit the essential oils that healthy individuals produce. This leads to extreme dryness and cracking, which can subsequently cause infection.

Cardiovascular Complications

Diabetes complications also include coronary artery disease and other cardiovascular problems. When blood sugar levels remain elevated on a constant basis, as is the case with certain diabetics, irreversible damage to the coronary arteries can occur. High blood sugar levels can also cause the individual's blood vessels to narrow or completely close, resulting in a heart attack or stroke, which typically come without warning. A link exists between coronary artery disease and obesity as well, as a diet high in sugar and fat often results in elevated cholesterol levels. High cholesterol may cause plaque buildup inside the arteries, which narrows the blood vessels. Exercising and taking a daily aspirin under a doctor's supervision can help to prevent these complications.

Nephropathy

Kidney problems, such as nephropathy are sometimes seen in long-term diabetics. Kidney tissue is made from thousands of tiny structures referred to as nephrons. These structures are responsible for removing waste from the human bloodstream. However, when nephrons are consistently bathed in glucose, as is the case with diabetics, they may thicken and develop scar tissue. This causes the kidneys to leak albumin (a protein) which eventually passes into the urine. Although not everyone with diabetes will experience this problem, those who smoke and obese individuals are at a higher than average risk for nephropathy. Keeping one's diabetes under control is the only way to prevent kidney problems.

Retinopathy

According to the American Diabetes Association, diabetes complications also include vision problems. This is because damage to small blood vessels is common in those afflicted with high blood sugar. Once the blood vessels become inflamed, blood flow to the eyes is reduced, leading to a disorder called retinopathy. In its early stages, weakened blood vessels develop small bulges that have the potential to eventually burst and leak into the retina of the eye. This can cause scar tissue to form, which may pull on the retina in the future, ultimately resulting in retinal detachment. If this occurs, vision loss is a serious threat. Regular eye exams and screenings are a diabetic's best line of defense against this complication.

Skin Disorders

Among the most common diabetes complications are skin disorders. Digital sclerosis and diabetic dermopathy are the top two skin conditions associated with high blood sugar, and both occur as a result of changes to the vessels that supply blood to the skin. Dermopathy presents as shiny, oval or round lesions, typically on the legs. Pain is not usually an issue, although the patches may be itchy at times. Digital sclerosis is a skin disorder characterized by the thickening and tightening of the skin on the hands and feet.

Those with type I--juvenile--diabetes may also be at high risk for a skin problem referred to as vitiligo. This condition is associated with an uneven complexion, due to the cells responsible for pigmentation being destroyed as a side effect of chronically high sugar levels. Vitiligo most often affects the stomach and chest, but can also appear on the face.

Risk of Infection

According to the National Institutes of Health, diabetics are at a greater risk for infections than healthy individuals. This is because high blood glucose levels suppress the immune system, making it more difficult for the person to fight off germs and bacteria. Of all the diabetes complications, infections are the most preventable, as there are many avenues through which to boost the human immune system. For example, consuming foods that are rich in antioxidants is an easy way to strengthen one's immunity and prevent certain illnesses. In addition, exercising on a regular basis can also bolster the immune system.

Because diabetes complications vary greatly from one patient to the next, it is important to discuss risk factors and preventative strategies with your physician. In this way, you can be sure you are doing everything possible to prevent such complications.

CHAPTER THREE

Healthy Lifestyles to Manage Type 2 Diabetes

Many people have lived with type 2 diabetes for a long and productive life. Some even have cured the disease. What are their secrets? An important takeaway from their success stories is that healthy lifestyles matter when dealing with diabetes. Eating healthy food, exercising regularly, and losing weight are all critical for blood sugar improvement. Through due diligence with healthy habits and medication, you can control and even reverse diabetes.

Monitor Blood Glucose Levels Everyday

Monitoring your blood glucose levels is essential to treat and heal type 2 diabetes. Checking your blood sugar is the only way you can know whether you are making progress and how food intake and exercise are affecting your blood sugar. It gives you a sense of accomplishment when you see the numbers within the normal range. Importantly, blood glucose tests can reveal dangerously high or low sugar levels.

Your doctor will determine how often you should check your blood glucose levels. With type 2 diabetes your doctor will typically recommend checking at least once a day determined by the amount of insulin doses taken each day. The best time for monitoring your blood sugar is in the morning before you eat or drink anything. That is the most precise reading, and it gives you a clear view of what has been going on during the night. If you are taking insulin injection, recommended testing times include before and after meals, and after fasting for 8 hours or longer. Managing the disease without insulin might not require daily checks.

Testing is done with a blood glucose meter, which has many different models available. Whether you have been given a blood glucose meter, or you have bought one yourself, they all work the same way. A meter includes a needle that is for pricking your skin, and strips for analyzing the blood. The process of testing is simple:

1) Make sure to wash your hands before pricking your finger.

2) Insert the strip into your meter, as instructed.

3) With the needle, prick the side of your fingertip.

4) Touch the strip with your finger, leaving the blood drop onto it.

5) Wait for your results to appear on the display.

6) Read the results.

According to the American Diabetes Association, following is normal ranges of blood glucose levels:

• Before meals, 80 - 130 milligrams per deciliter (mg/dL)

• 1-2 Hours after the start of meals, below 180 mg/dL

An important part of testing is to log daily results along with your daily diet and exercise regimen. Bring this record to your doctor visits to monitor your progress of recovery. There are printable records available online to help with daily recording.

Lose Weight and Exercise Regularly

Approximately 90% of people with type 2 diabetes are carrying extra pounds. In fact, overweight can lead to a worsening condition known as insulin resistance. Too much fat in the body can interfere with the function of insulin that is necessary for the body to process glucose. If you are overweight and suffer from type 2 diabetes, weight loss can improve your body's response to insulin and lower blood sugar. The American Diabetes Association has concluded that just losing 10 to 15 pounds will significantly lower blood sugar levels.

Eating healthy foods and regular exercise are proven ways to lose weight and keep it off. We have addressed eating healthy foods in previous sections of the book, and will now discuss the importance of physical exercise.

Regular aerobic or cardio exercise is good for cardiovascular health and helps burning calories. Getting aerobic exercise at least three times per week for 20 minutes a time is an excellent way to extend stamina. You could use a cardio machine such as an elliptical, stationary bike, or a treadmill. You could also walk, jog, hike, swim, bike or run.

Strength training helps increase body's lean muscle mass. Because it takes more energy to maintain muscle than fat, people who build muscle mass will burn a higher number of calories than people who have less muscle. Even when sedentary, more calories must be burned to support a muscular body than a body with poor muscle tone and excess fat. Toning your body at least three times a week using a stability ball, dumbbells, or a resistance band for 15-20 minutes at a time will have a significant impact.

If exercising sounds like a daunting task now, know that it doesn't have to be. There isn't a strict path you should follow. Try as many different exercises as you like, combine or modify some, get creative and invent some new ways that will keep you active and your body mass in check, and take control over diabetes.

When you start new exercise activities or increase workout intensities, remember to track blood glucose levels before, during and after a workout. Blood glucose tests not only show you how your body is improving but also help to prevent dangerous blood glucose fluctuations. Excessive physical activities may lead to hypoglycemia, which is defined by blood glucose levels below 70 mg/dL. Hypoglycemia may cause nausea, weakness, unconsciousness and accident, and should be avoided.

If you are taking diabetes medications or insulin, make sure that you measure blood glucose before exercise. After 30 minutes of exercise, check blood glucose level again. If your blood glucose level is lower than 100 mg/dL, take a break, eat some fruits or snacks, and carry on if you feel up to it. Stop exercising if your blood glucose level is lower than 70 mg/dL, or if you feel short of breath, pain or shaky.

If you plan on beginning any new diet or exercise plans to lose weight, speak with your doctor to make sure that the food choices, meal planning, and workout intensities are the right fit for you.

Limit Alcohol Consumption

For all of you who enjoy a glass of wine over dinner, here is some good news – alcohol is not off limits when you have diabetes, especially if you have your sugar levels under control. The American Diabetes Association recommends no more than one alcoholic drink per day for women and no more than two drinks a day for men (1 drink = 12 ounces of beer = 5 ounces of wine = 1.5 ounces of liquor).

The reason to limit alcohol intake is that alcohol can increase the risks of diabetes complications. What are these risks?

Hypoglycemia – is when your blood glucose levels fall too low. Drinking alcohol can increase the chances of this happening, especially if you're on insulin or certain types of medication. Why does this happen? Usually, when your blood glucose levels drop, your liver will convert the carbohydrates that it stored, into glucose – keeping your sugar levels stable and preventing hypoglycemia.

When you have alcohol in your system, your liver's priority is to remove the alcohol from your body. The presence of alcohol inhibits liver's capacity of producing glucose, leading to hypoglycemia. Hypoglycemia causes dizziness and disorientation, so it can make you seem like you are drunk. It is best always to carry an ID that says you are diabetic, to get the right treatment if such time comes.

If you're diabetic, and you drank alcohol, check your blood glucose level before you sleep. If it's in the range of 100 to 140 mg/dL, you're fine. If it's lower than that, eat something. If you do drink alcohol, make sure to eat foods with carbohydrates to prevent hypoglycemia.

High Blood Pressure is a complication of diabetes that should be a cause for concern. Regularly consuming significant amounts of alcohol can raise your blood pressure, causing other conditions such as cardiovascular disease.

Neuropathy is another complication of diabetes which can be exacerbated by alcohol. It is linked to high blood pressure and is a condition where your nerves are damaged.

Weight Gain is possible due to the high-calorie content of alcoholic drinks. Since diabetics are being advised to lose weight, drinking alcohol doesn't help.

Here are some tips for alcohol consumption:
- Never drink on an empty stomach.
- Do not drive within a couple of hours after consuming an alcoholic drink.
- Have a glass of water with you to keep you hydrated. Switch to water after your first drink.
- Drink slowly.
- If you can avoid alcohol altogether, you'll be doing yourself a big favor!

Quit Smoking

According to the Centers for Disease Control and Prevention, smokers are 30-40% more likely to develop type 2 diabetes. Smoking makes it harder to manage blood sugar levels and increases the chances of developing complications. Smoking is bad enough for non-diabetics, but for those who are already diabetic, it can be a catalyst to complications such as cardiovascular diseases, kidney disease, neuropathy, and retinopathy.

It can be quite a nerve-wracking process to stop something you have been doing for so long, but there are many 'tools' that will help you quit smoking. You might be tempted to toss away cigarettes and quit smoking once and for all. However, many people who try to stop smoking suddenly without any form of therapy wind up relapsing. Without a cigarette, the body will go through the nicotine withdrawal symptoms, which include a headache, drowsiness, and anxiety. Nicotine gums, patches, and electronic cigarettes may help minimize nicotine withdrawal symptoms.

Don't quit smoking all by yourself. Tell your family and even your friends on social networks about your plan to stop smoking. Their encouragement will help you succeed. One of the reasons that people smoke is to relieve stress. If you are planning on quitting, you need new ways to deal with stress. Yoga, meditation, and listening to music can help you reduce stress.

Prevent Complications

While diabetes complications seem to be an inevitable part of this disease, they can be very well prevented. Taking a proper care of yourself and monitor the warning signs can help you avoid serious threats to your health.

Taking Care of Your Feet

High blood glucose can cause severe damage to your feet when you have diabetes. Your feet are prone to:

• Poor circulation. Due to the disease blood vessels in the legs and feet narrow and harden, which causes a poor flow of the blood.

• Foot ulcers. When you have a foot ulcer, your high glucose levels can only complicate things and make it hard for the ulcer to heal and may contribute to developing an infection. In severe cases, toe, foot or leg amputations are necessary to stop the infection.

• Calluses. When you have diabetes, you are prone to building up calluses in high-pressure feet areas.

• Skin damage. Diabetes can dry and crack the skin on your feet.

It is of great importance that you see a podiatrist once a year. You can take good care of your feet by:

• Washing your feet with warm water and soap each day, and keeping them clean and dry. Because many diabetics are insensitive to heat, care must be taken to test the water temperature before immersing one's feet.

• Wearing comfortable shoes that do not pinch your toes and feet. Shoes that don't fit can cause calluses, nail problems, and ulcers.

• Wearing diabetic socks or antithrombotic stockings, both of which significantly increase circulation in the feet.

• Never walking barefoot and avoiding sitting with your legs crossed.

• Inspecting your feet on a daily basis, and regularly trimming your nails to a comfortable length. Due to insensitivity, it is possible for a person to step on a sharp object or not feel something in his or her shoe, which can lead to long-term foot damage.

• Treating ulcers and wounds urgently.

Taking Care of Your Eyes

Diabetes complications also include vision problems. This is because damage to small blood vessels is common in diabetics. Once the blood vessels become inflamed, blood flow to the eyes is reduced, leading to a disorder called retinopathy that may eventually lead to blindness. It is, therefore, crucial that you see an ophthalmologist for a regular eye examination, at least once a year. It is important to visit your doctor if:

- Your vision is blurred
- You feel pressure in your eyes
- Your eyes have turned red
- You have watering eyes
- You see flashes of light
- You see dark spots

Avoiding Gastroparesis

Gastroparesis is a common condition that affects people with diabetes, and it is a delayed gastric emptying. Besides the obvious complications of this disorder, gastroparesis makes it harder for diabetics to manage their glucose levels. To avoid this, it is recommended for diabetics to:

- Eat slowly.
- Sit upright during meals.
- Take a walk after meals.

Following are the common signs of gastroparesis:
- Vomiting
- Heartburn
- Nausea
- Lack of appetite
- Abdominal bloating

If you fear you may be affected by this condition, seek medical help immediately.

Relax

Stress can negatively affect insulin levels and make it hard to manage blood glucose levels. When you're stressed, the stress hormones epinephrine and cortisol kick in. Their role is to raise blood sugar levels for energy when you need it the most. This is good for emergencies like when you need to run away from a hungry lion that's chasing you – but certainly not good for raising blood sugar constantly.

Learn to manage your stress. It may be hard at first since we live in a fast-paced society. Use these simple tips to relieve stress.

• Start doing things that make you happy – playing a musical instrument, doing an art task, fishing, reading a book you enjoy, or spending the morning in the garden.

• Try yoga and exercise. The combination of relaxing yoga poses and deep breathing techniques helps reduce the levels of cortisol in the blood and lower blood pressure. In addition to its health benefits mentioned earlier, exercise also triggers the release of the hormone endorphin that relieves stress. Outdoor exercise and walking along a nature trail can be highly meditative and do wonders for your health.

• Mindfulness. Being mindful means being in the present, fully aware and observing things without judgment. For instance, when you walk down the street, try to be in the present: listen to the chirping of the birds, feel how the wind gently tickles your skin, focus on people's chattering, etc. Try to be mindful all the time, whether you are stuck in the traffic, or at a meeting. It will help you relax, and you will learn to deal with stressful situations without letting them get the best of you.

• Meditation. We all know the benefits of this ancient technique, but what makes it ideal for people with diabetes is the fact that it reduces stress, slows the heart rate, and achieves balance. You do not need to meditate like a monk, and you can start with taking deep breaths at a quiet place. Purchase a book on meditation for beginners or buy a DVD, that will help you master this amazing relaxing technique.

• Do things that make use of your talents. For example, if you are excellent with your hands, then create things for yourself, your family or friends. If you like animals, think about owning a pet.

• Go out to a movie or dinner with friends.

• Spend time with persons who make you feel happy about yourself – individuals who treat you well. Keep away from people who treat you poorly.

What's imperative is that you unwind and keep stress from building up.

Sleep Well

Diabetics often have poor sleeping patterns, and this can make their blood glucose levels harder to control. In a 1999 Lancet study completed at the University of Chicago, researchers found that diabetics who got only four hours of sleep a night, for a week, had impaired glucose tolerance. If you have diabetes, it is important to get at least seven to eight hours of sleep each day. Chronic sleep deprivation raises the hormone cortisol which promotes insulin resistance.

Research has shown that sleep deprivation reduced the levels of the hormone leptin, and at the same time increased the levels of the hormone Ghrelin. Leptin is an appetite suppressant, and Ghrelin is an appetite stimulant. When your appetite is stimulated by sleep deprivation, you will crave for foods high in carbohydrates and fats. This will not help your goal of losing the extra weight.

Bedroom Environment

To sleep better at night, create a sleep-splendid space in your bedroom. Remove any televisions, gaming systems, computers, or other electronics from that room, and make it a space that invites rest. Keep the room cool, ideally between 60 and 67 degrees. There shouldn't be any distracting noise. White noise or background noise such as a fan or a water element can be helpful.

Check your lighting. You want total darkness when you're trying to sleep, so hang some curtains at any windows or doors where light might leak in. The end result should be an oasis of calm.

You may need to make some adjustments to your bed. Make sure your mattress and pillows are comfortable and clean. If you've been sleeping in the same bed for 10 years or more, it might be time to invest in a new and more supportive mattress. There are a number of them on the market designed to help consumers sleep better.

Bedtime Rituals

You can improve your chances of getting a good night's sleep by establishing and sticking to a regular routine. Even if you consider yourself impulsive and spontaneous, your body appreciates a routine and responds to it. Set up a bedtime schedule. Try to go to bed and wake up at the same time every night, even on the weekends or when you don't have to work or get up early. This will set your internal clock and help you get into a pattern of sleeping at regular times.

Train your body to know it's bedtime. Take a warm bath or shower, or do something specific that separates your awake activities to your bedtime activities. Read a book for a little while, sip some chamomile tea, or listen to some relaxing music. Establishing these rituals will help you transition into sleep.

Many diabetics have sleep apnea, restless legs syndrome and peripheral neuropathy, which can interfere with their sleep.

Sleep Apnea is when you pause breathing while you sleep. It is caused by an obstruction of the upper airway. Sleep apnea prompts the brain to wake you up. This keeps you from having a deep and satisfying sleep.

There are many available treatments for sleep apnea. The doctor may recommend that you lose some weight if you are overweight. Another solution is to wear a mask over your nose. This treatment is called CPAP or continuous positive airway pressure. It keeps your airways from closing while you sleep. It's a temporary solution, not a cure.

Restless Legs Syndrome is the feeling that you need to move your legs, for several reasons. You may feel tingling, pain, burning and numbness. It's a type of sleeping disorder common to diabetics and can be treated with pain relievers, sleeping aids and dopamine agents.

Peripheral Neuropathy has the same symptoms as restless legs syndrome and can make it difficult to go to sleep and stay asleep.

If you have sleep apnea or other sleep disorders, consult with your doctor and get treatment.

Plan Your Trips Well

Without careful planning, travel can disrupt your diabetic diet and treatment plan, and spell trouble. When you travel, you may be forced to eat fast foods that are high in sugar and fat. It is possible that your prescription medicine is not available in the places that you are going to.

Following are some tips to keep you safe and on track.

Doctor's visit. Before you go, visit your doctor and tell him/her about your trip plan, and ask for extra prescriptions. Have him/her examine you to make sure that you are safe to travel. Ask him to write a letter that will help you in the case of emergencies; the letter should explain your condition, say what medications you need to take, as well as list allergies or other medicaments you may be sensitive to.

Prepare for an emergency. When traveling in a foreign country (especially if you travel somewhere where English is not the first language) you need to be prepared in case of emergency. Check the IAMAT (International Association for Medical Assistance to Travelers) for a list of English-speaking doctors.

Pack. Packing for your trip is the first and the most important thing, as you need to make sure that you haven't forgotten any necessary items:

• Have your medical ID with you at all times. Write 'I have diabetes' also in another language if needed.

• Have your medical supplies close to you. Pack the insulin and syringes, (if you take insulin shots) you may need some cold pack in an insulated bag for those medications that go in the fridge (like insulin). Do not forget your glucose meter, strips and lancets.

• All of the other medications. This is important especially if you're going to a secluded location where you might not find a drugstore that carries your medicine.

• Bring some healthy snacks and extra candy in case your blood sugar levels fall sharply.

• Bring a first aid kit.

Call the airline and inquire about special meals, if you're taking a long trip. In the airport, you can inform the authorities that you are diabetic and carrying medications. If you're wearing an insulin pump, let them know. Make sure you have your prescription on hand and that they are properly labeled.

Adjust to different time zones. If you take insulin shots, do not forget to plan the time of the injections well.

When you arrive:

• Do not drink tap water. Always have a bottle of water with you.

• Do not go barefoot. Yes, not even on the beach.

• Take along snacks, especially when you go sightseeing. Your blood sugar may go low, so you will need something that will increase the glucose levels. A banana always helps.

• Check your blood sugar regularly.

CHAPTER FOUR

Diabetic Diet

Once you're a diabetic, your choice of food will directly affect the results of your diabetes management program, which involves the following:

- taking the right medication regularly;
- monitoring blood glucose levels;
- having an active lifestyle; and
- going on a diabetes diet.

Of all of the above, the mention of a diabetes diet instantly elicits a negative response from diabetics who already may feel deprived and depressed. This is understandable, since food is a source of comfort and gratification for us humans. Not only do we need to eat, but we love to eat.

Is going on a diabetes diet as bad as it sounds? What does that mean anyway?

A diabetes diet is not a condemnation to a lifetime of bland and tasteless food—it simply means eating foods that are low in carbohydrates and added sugar, low in fat, low in sodium, high in nutrition, high in protein, and moderate to low in calories.

What do you think? Are you still thinking that means a piece of cardboard served on a plate? That's the usual reaction. At the mention of all of these "lows," diabetics fear they may never enjoy food again. It's a sad thought, but one that is totally baseless. Before I tell you why you don't need to be sad and feel deprived, I'd like to share with you the WHY of the diabetes diet. Why do you need to lower your intake of sugar, carbohydrates, salt, and fats? Why do you need to lose weight? Once you know why you need to watch what you eat and drink, you will be more motivated and have the determination to stick to your program.

Why Should You Limit Your Carbohydrate Intake?

To lower blood sugar levels, you should limit carbohydrate intake. Carbs become sugar and sugar must be avoided as much as possible. Since we need carbohydrates for energy, it is not advised that you remove them from your diet entirely. A balanced diet is preferable to ensure you're getting all of the sustenance you need.

Diabetics should aim for 45 to 60 grams of carbohydrates per meal and 15 to 30 grams for snacks. Choose complex carbohydrates found in beans, whole grains, and vegetables instead of simple carbohydrates, such as sugar and corn syrup. Since people respond to carbohydrates differently, the best way to know if you are getting too much is to test yourself after each meal. Count the carbs in your food to see how much it affects your blood sugar levels. To further integrate carbohydrate monitoring into your diabetes treatment, a dietitian can help set specific goals for carbohydrates to be included in each meal and snack.

Why You Should Avoid Sugar

If a diabetic is advised to limit carbohydrates because they turn to sugar, it follows that sugar itself should be avoided. Sodas, candies, sports drinks, fruit drinks—all of these beverages will catapult your sugar levels to unwanted heights, not to mention that they contain a lot of calories.

To give you an example: one can of regular soda contains around 10 teaspoons of sugar and 150 calories. When you think about how much soda a regular person consumes in one sitting, it's no wonder we've become sugar addicts.

The World Health Organization initially set the recommended daily intake of sugar to 10% of your total calories—that's 200 calories. In their latest recommendation, they've lowered it further to just 5%, equivalent to 100 calories. As one teaspoon of sugar is

16 calories, you are technically only allowed six teaspoons of sugar a day, way less than what we're used to consuming.

Not only does sugar raise your blood glucose levels, it can also cause fatty liver, which is common among diabetics. In a recent study by the US Centers for Disease Control and Prevention, it was concluded that large amounts of additional sugar in a diet increases the risk of heart disease by as much as 30%.

Sugar is hard to avoid because not only is it delicious, but most food labels hide the sugar content. Anything that ends in "ose" is sugar-related, including high-fructose corn syrup (HFCS), caramel, treacle, malt syrup, maltodextrine, fruit concentrate, and more. The good news is that there are many sugar-free alternatives available nowadays.

Why Fruits and Vegetables are Good for Diabetics

For people dealing with diabetes, a plant-based diet is the best option for their health. This means filling your plate with fruits and vegetables. The reason fruits and vegetables work so well for the diabetes diet is that they are packed with vitamins, minerals, and other nutrients. They are low in fat and calories, and the fiber they contain helps slow down the absorption of glucose in the body.

Five portions—roughly what will fit in your palm—is the recommended amount of daily fruits and vegetables.

Large, healthy salads are always a good choice. Add flavor by topping salads with protein like chicken, tuna, or shrimp. Sprinkle it with nuts and seeds and enjoy a homemade dressing made with olive oil, vinegar, and your favorite spices. Fruit makes an excellent snack when you're craving something sweet, especially berries, apples, and cantaloupe.

When you're planning meals or looking for a snack, make sure that at least half of your plate is covered with a combination of fruits and vegetables. Combined with whole grains and low-fat protein sources, you'll create a healthy, balanced diet that allows you to lower your blood sugar, protect your heart, and feel a lot better.

Diabetes Superfoods

Studies have shown that some vegetables and spices are especially helpful in lowering blood sugar. These diabetes superfoods include celery, bitter melon, pumpkin, tomatoes, spinach, beans, berries, nuts, and cinnamon. These superfoods can improve the body's sensitivity to insulin, repair damaged cells in the pancreas, and reduce blood sugar levels.

Cut Back on Saturated Fats and Avoid Trans Fats

Everybody needs dietary fats to remain healthy. Because fats have higher calorie counts than carbohydrates and proteins, try to eat high-fat foods in moderation. Diabetics should watch the consumption of saturated fats and avoid trans fats.

Saturated Fats

One of the complications of diabetes is heart disease. Studies have shown that high saturated fat consumption increases the levels of LDL (bad cholesterol) while reduces the levels of HDL (good cholesterol), leading to plaque formation and clogging of arteries. Being a diabetic, you are already at a greater risk for a heart disease, so it is important to consume saturated fats in moderation.

Foods High in Saturated Fats:
- Butter
- Lard
- Chocolate

- Coconut and Coconut Oil
- Cream Sauces
- Palm Oil

Saturated fats are also found in fried foods, processed foods, red meats, hot dogs, high-fat dairy products, and poultry skin. In Nutrition Fact labels, saturated fats are listed under total fats.

Trans Fats

Just like saturated fats, trans fats raise bad cholesterol and reduce good cholesterol in the blood. Many studies have shown that trans fats have more severe effects on heart health than even saturated fats. So avoid trans fats entirely.

Most trans fats are produced artificially by the food industry that hydrogenates vegetable oils to increase their shelf life and to enhance the flavor of processed foods. Trans fats are by-products of the oil hydrogenation process. Trans fats can be found in processed foods, cookies, baked goods, cream pies, margarine, shortening and fried foods from some restaurants. When shopping for groceries, double check the trans-fat section in the Nutrition Facts labels, and avoid those foods containing partially hydrogenated or hydrogenated vegetable oils. If a particular food contains 0.5 grams of trans fats the label will most likely say 0 grams. That is why it is a good idea to check the list of the ingredients.

Healthy Fats

Instead of saturated fats and trans fats, choose monounsaturated fats and polyunsaturated fats. These healthy fats can be found in the following foods.

Foods High in Monosaturated Fats
- Avocados
- Olive oil
- Sesame Seeds

• Peanut Oil
• Almonds
• Cashews

Foods High in Polyunsaturated Fats
• Walnuts
• Pumpkin Seeds
• Sunflower Seeds
• Soybean Oil
• Corn Oil
• Cottonseed Oil

Omega-3 fatty acids are polyunsaturated fatty acids that your body needs for normal functions. Omega-3 fatty acids can protect the heart by lowering the levels of cholesterol and triglycerides in the blood, by reducing blood pressure, and by suppressing inflammation.

Foods Rich in Omega 3 Fatty Acids
• Salmon
• Sardines
• Mackerel
• Trout
• Herring
• Flaxseeds

Why Cut Back on Sodium?

A high-sodium diet also causes high-blood pressure. Similar to the reason why you should cut down on fats, you should also reduce the salt in your food. Diabetics should aim for only 2300 mg of sodium or less daily. Studies have shown that approximately 75% of the sodium in an average American's diet comes from processed and packaged foods.

Eating fresh and unprocessed foods is the easiest way to ensure your sodium intake meets the daily allowance, without putting yourself at a higher risk for heart attack or stroke.

CHAPTER FIVE

Diabetic Recipes

The 28 healthy and delicious recipes in this chapter are diabetic-friendly. Enjoy these breakfast, lunch, snack, and dinner recipes while familiarizing yourself with the diabetes diet.

Breakfast

Scrambled Eggs with Mushroom and Spinach

Yield: 2 servings
Ingredients:
2 eggs, large
2 egg whites
⅛ teaspoon salt
⅛ teaspoon pepper
1 teaspoon butter
½ cup fresh mushrooms, sliced thin
½ cup fresh baby spinach (or your favorite green veggie), chopped
2 tablespoons shredded parmesan cheese

Directions:
1. Beat eggs, egg whites, pepper, and salt in a bowl until thoroughly mixed.
2. Using a small, nonstick skillet, heat the butter over low-medium heat. Cook the mushrooms, stirring as you cook for 3–4 minutes or until tender.
3. Add spinach. Cook until slightly wilted. Lower heat.

4. Add beaten egg mixture and stir until eggs are thickened and thoroughly cooked. Stir in cheese.

Nutritional Information (Per Serving)
Calories: 134
Fat: 8.5 g
Sat Fat: 3.8 g
Carbohydrates: 1.8 g
Fiber: 0.4 g
Sugar: 1 g
Protein: 12.9 g
Sodium: 336 mg

Tomato and Zucchini Omelet

Yield: 4 servings
Ingredients:
⅓ cup sun-dried tomatoes
1½ cups egg substitute
½ cup cottage cheese
2 green onions, chopped
¼ cup minced fresh basil or 1 tablespoon dried basil
⅛ teaspoon crushed red pepper flakes
1 cup fresh broccoli
1 cup zucchini, sliced
1 medium red pepper, chopped
2 teaspoons canola oil
1 cup boiling water
2 tablespoons Parmesan cheese, grated

Directions:
1. Place the tomatoes in a bowl and cover with boiling water. Let stand for 5 minutes. Drain and put aside.

2. In another bowl, mix the egg substitute, onions, basil, pepper flakes, cottage cheese, and tomatoes. Set aside.

3. In a 10-inch oven-proof skillet, sauté the zucchini, red pepper, and broccoli in oil until tender. Lower heat and top with the egg mixture. Cover and cook for 4–6 minutes or until nearly set.

4. Sprinkle with Parmesan cheese, then heat for 2 minutes or until eggs are completely set. Let sit for 5 minutes. Cut into wedges and serve.

Nutritional Information (Per Serving)
Calories: 135
Fat: 3.9 g
Sat Fat: 1 g
Carbohydrates: 7.6 g
Fiber: 1.7 g

Sugar: 3.6 g
Protein: 17.9 g
Sodium: 342 mg

Spinach and Onion Scramble

Yield: 4 servings
Ingredients:
6 eggs
1 tablespoon almond milk
6 ounces fresh baby spinach
1 cup red onion, chopped
2 garlic cloves, minced
1 tablespoon olive oil
Salt and pepper to taste

Directions:
1. Heat the olive oil in a skillet over medium heat. Add the garlic and onion, and cook for 3 minutes.

2. Add the spinach and heat until it begins to wilt.

3. While the vegetables are cooking, beat the eggs and the almond milk together.

4. Add the egg mixture to the pan and scramble all ingredients together until the eggs are cooked.

5. Serve with salt and pepper.

Nutritional Information (Per Serving)
Calories: 157
Fat: 11.2 g
Sat Fat: 3.4 g
Carbohydrates: 5.5 g
Fiber: 1.7 g
Sugar: 2.1 g
Protein: 10 g

Carrot Bread

Yield: 8 servings

Ingredients:

2 cups almond flour

1 teaspoon baking powder

1 tablespoon cumin seeds

Salt to taste

3 large eggs

2 tablespoons olive oil

1 tablespoon apple cider vinegar

3 cups carrots, peeled and grated

½ teaspoon fresh ginger, peeled and grated finely

¼ cup raisins

Directions:

1. Preheat your oven to 350 degrees F.

2. Line a loaf pan with parchment paper.

3. In a large bowl, add almond flour, baking powder, cumin seeds, and salt and mix well.

4. In another bowl, add the eggs, olive oil, and vinegar, and beat until well combined.

5. Add egg mixture to the flour mixture, and mix until well combined.

6. Gently fold in carrot, ginger, and raisins.

7. Place the mixture into the prepared loaf pan.

8. Bake for about 1 hour until a toothpick inserted in the center comes out clean.

Nutritional Information (Per Serving)

Calories: 255

Fat: 19.4 g

Sat Fat: 2.1 g

Carbohydrates: 15.3 g

Fiber: 4.6 g

Sugar: 6.4 g
Protein: 9.1 g

Mushroom Muffins

Yield: 6 servings
Ingredients:
1 teaspoon olive oil
1½ cups fresh mushrooms, chopped
1 scallion, chopped
1 teaspoon garlic, minced
1 teaspoon fresh rosemary, minced
Freshly ground black pepper to taste
1 (12.3-ounce) package lite, firm, silken tofu, drained
¼ cup unsweetened soy milk
2 tablespoons nutritional yeast
1 tablespoon arrowroot starch
1 teaspoon unsalted butter, softened
¼ teaspoon ground turmeric

Directions:
1. Preheat oven to 375 degrees F. Grease a 12-cup muffin pan.
2. In a nonstick skillet, heat oil on medium heat.
3. Add scallion and garlic and sauté for about 1 minute.
4. Add mushrooms and sauté for about 5–7 minutes.
5. Stir in rosemary and black pepper and remove from the heat.
6. Keep aside to cool slightly.
7. In a food processor, add tofu and remaining ingredients and pulse until smooth.
8. Transfer tofu mixture into a large bowl.
9. Fold in mushroom mixture.
10. Spoon mixture evenly into prepared muffin cups.

11. Bake for about 20–22 minutes or until a toothpick inserted in center comes out clean.

12. Remove muffin pan from oven and place on wire rack to cool for about 10 minutes.

13. Carefully, invert muffins onto wire rack and serve warm.

Nutritional Information (Per Serving)
Calories: 88
Fat: 4.2 g
Sat Fat: 1 g
Carbohydrates: 7.3 g
Fiber: 1.4 g
Sugar: 1.9 g
Protein: 7.2 g
Sodium: 21 mg

Tapioca Pancakes

Yield: 6 servings
Ingredients:
½ cup tapioca flour
½ cup almond flour
½ teaspoon red chili powder
¼ teaspoon salt
Black pepper to taste
1 cup coconut milk
½ red onion, chopped
¼ teaspoon fresh ginger, minced
1 serrano pepper, seeded and minced
½ cup fresh parsley leaves, chopped
2 tablespoons olive oil

Directions:
1. In a large bowl, mix together flours and spices. Add the coconut milk, and mix until well combined.

2. Fold in the onion, ginger, serrano pepper, and cilantro.

3. Lightly grease a large nonstick skillet with oil, and heat over medium heat.

4. Add about ¼ cup of mixture, and tilt the pan to spread it evenly in the skillet. Cook for about 3–4 minutes for both sides.

5. Repeat with the remaining mixture.

6. Serve with your desired topping.

Nutritional Information (Per Serving)
Calories: 146
Fat: 10.1 g
Sat Fat: 1.8 g
Carbohydrates: 13.1 g
Fiber: 1.4 g
Sugar: 1.4 g
Protein: 2.4 g

Sodium: 107 mg

Multigrain Hot Cereal

Yield: 8 servings
Ingredients:
½ cup pearl barley
½ cup red wheat berries
½ cup brown rice
¼ cup steel cut oats
3 tablespoons quinoa
¼ teaspoon kosher salt
1½ quarts water

Directions:

1. Add all ingredients to a saucepan, stir to mix and bring to a boil.

2. Reduce the heat to low and allow to simmer for 45 minutes giving it an occasional stir.

3. The cereal can be refrigerated and reheated for quick breakfasts or snacks throughout the week.

Nutritional Information (Per Serving)
Calories: 118
Fat: 1.0 g
Sat Fat: 0 g
Carbohydrates: 23.6 g
Fiber: 4.3 g
Sugar: 0.6 g
Protein: 4.0 g
Sodium: 74.6 mg

Lunch

Roasted Celery Root with Baby Carrots

Yield: 4 servings

Ingredients:

1 pound celery root, diced into 1-inch squares
2 teaspoons olive oil
1 small pinch of black pepper
2 inch-long sprigs of fresh rosemary
½ pound baby carrots

Directions:

1. Preheat the oven to 375 degrees F.

2. Place diced celery root in a medium bowl and add 1 teaspoon of olive oil, black pepper, and rosemary. Toss until celery root is fully coated before placing into baking dish.

3. Bake in the oven for 45 minutes, until golden brown.

4. Place the carrots in a medium bowl and add 1 teaspoon of olive oil. Toss until carrots are fully coated. Put the mixture in a baking dish and bake in the oven for 30 minutes. (This can be started 15 minutes after celery root had been put into oven in order to ensure equal cooking time.)

5. Once both dishes have been baked, combine in a large serving bowl and serve while hot.

Nutritional Information (Per Serving)
Calories: 88
Fat: 2.8 g
Sat Fat: 0.4 g
Carbohydrates: 15.2 g
Fiber: 3.7 g
Sugar: 4.5 g
Protein: 2.1 g
Sodium: 158 mg

Spinach Salad with Shrimp

Yield: 3 servings
Ingredients:
4 tablespoons olive oil
3 tablespoons red wine vinegar
1 tablespoon spicy mustard
1 garlic clove, minced
Salt and pepper to taste
1 cup small salad shrimp, cooked and chilled
12 ounces fresh baby spinach
½ cup grape tomatoes, halved
¼ cup sliced red onion
½ cup sliced mushrooms
¼ cup chopped walnuts

Directions:
1. In a bowl, whisk together the oil, vinegar, mustard, garlic, salt, and pepper. Add the shrimp and toss until it's all coated.

2. In a large bowl, toss together the spinach, tomatoes, onion, and mushrooms.

3. Add the shrimp to the bowl and toss everything together.

4. Top with the walnuts.

Nutritional Information (Per Serving)
Calories: 400
Fat: 27.2 g
Sat Fat: 3.7 g
Carbohydrates: 10.7 g
Fiber: 3.9 g
Sugar: 3.1 g
Protein: 31.1 g

Green Bean and Anchovy Salad

Yield: 3 servings

Ingredients:

1 pound fresh green beans

1 can anchovies, rinsed

2 cloves garlic, minced

¼ cup olive oil

Directions:

1. Rinse and trim the green beans.

2. Heat a pot of water until it's boiling. Add the green beans and cook for 5 minutes, then rinse.

3. In another pot, heat the olive oil and add the anchovies and the garlic. Use a wooden spoon to break down the anchovies until they dissolve into the oil.

4. Toss the anchovies and oil with the green beans.

Nutritional Information (Per Serving)

Calories: 225

Fat: 18.5 g

Sat Fat: 2.8 g

Carbohydrates: 11.4 g

Fiber: 5.2 g

Sugar: 2.1 g

Protein: 7.2 g

Sodium: 560 mg

Italian Antipasto Salad

Yield: 4 servings
Ingredients:
2 cups romaine lettuce, chopped
2 cups radicchio lettuce, chopped
½ cup marinated artichokes, chopped
½ cup mushrooms, chopped
1 stalk celery, chopped
½ red onion, sliced
1 cup grape tomatoes, chopped
¼ cup roasted red peppers, chopped
6 ounces mozzarella cheese, chopped
½ stick pepperoni, chopped
¼ cup olive oil
3 tablespoons balsamic vinegar

Directions:
1. Combine all the vegetables and top with the pepperoni and cheese.
2. Add the olive oil and the vinegar and toss together.

Nutritional Information (Per Serving)
Calories: 431
Fat: 34.2 g
Sat Fat: 11 g
Carbohydrates: 11.3 g
Fiber: 3.1 g
Sugar: 3.2 g
Protein: 21.8 g
Sodium: 845 mg

Fish and Squash Meal

Yield: 4 servings

Ingredients:

1 teaspoon grated lemon peel

1 red onion, chopped

1 cup zucchini, cut into squares

1 cup squash, cut into squares

1 teaspoon minced garlic

4 fish fillets, sliced 1 inch thick

2 tablespoons fresh mint leaves, finely chopped

1 tablespoon red wine vinegar

2 tablespoons extra virgin olive oil

1 tablespoon water

Directions:

1. Preheat oven to 400 degrees F.

2. In a baking dish, combine grated lemon, 1 tablespoon of oil, and onions. Spread on dish evenly. Bake in oven until onion is translucent for about 15 minutes, stirring occasionally.

3. Remove from oven. Add the zucchini, squash, and garlic and mix. Make sure it's spread evenly before returning to oven to bake for another 10 minutes.

4. Remove from oven once cooked.

5. Increase oven temperature to 450 degrees F. Move vegetables to one side and add fish fillets. Spoon vegetables over fish.

6. Return the dish to the oven and bake until fish is flaky, 10 minutes for thin fillets and 15 minutes for thicker fillets.

7. In a small bowl, combine remaining oil with vinegar, water, mint leaves, and onion.

5. Spoon the spice mixture over fillets and serve.

Nutritional Information (Per Serving)

Calories: 295
Fat: 18.3 g
Sat Fat: 3.6 g
Carbohydrates: 20.7 g
Fiber: 2 g
Sugar: 2.3 g
Protein: 14.5 g
Sodium: 493 mg

Balsamic Chicken and Beans

Yield: 4 servings

Ingredients:

4 skinless, boneless chicken breasts

¼ cup balsamic vinegar

2 garlic cloves, minced

2 shallots, sliced

3 tablespoons extra virgin olive oil

1 pound fresh green beans, trimmed

2 tablespoons red pepper flakes

Directions:

1. Combine 2 tablespoons of the olive oil with the balsamic vinegar, garlic, and shallots. Pour it over the chicken breasts and refrigerate overnight.

2. The next day, preheat the oven to 375 degrees F.

3. Take the chicken out of the marinade and arrange in a shallow baking pan. Discard the rest of the marinade.

3. Bake in the oven for 40 minutes.

4. While the chicken is cooking, bring a large pot of water to a boil. Place the green beans in the water and allow them to cook for five minutes and then drain.

5. Heat one tablespoon of olive oil in the pot and return the green beans after rinsing them. Toss with red pepper flakes.

Nutritional Information (Per Serving)

Calories: 433

Fat: 17.4 g

Sat Fat: 3.3 g

Carbohydrates: 12.9 g

Fiber: 4.6 g

Sugar: 3.1 g

Protein: 56.1 g

Sodium: 140 mg

Stuffed Chicken Breast

Yield: 4 servings
Ingredients:
4 (4-ounce) skinless, boneless chicken breast halves, pounded to ½-inch thickness
Pinch of salt
Freshly ground black pepper to taste
¼ cup Kalamata olives, pitted and chopped
¼ cup oil packed sun-dried tomatoes, drained
¼ cup feta cheese, crumbled
1 tablespoon fresh dill, chopped
1 tablespoon fresh parsley, chopped
1 tablespoon olive oil

Directions:
1. Preheat oven to 375 degrees F. Grease a rimmed baking sheet.
2. Rub chicken with pinch of salt and black pepper.
3. In a large bowl, mix olives, tomatoes, feta cheese, scallion, dill, and parsley.
4. Place chicken breast on cutting board.
5. Stuff chicken breasts with olive mixture and roll tightly.
6. Secure each roll with toothpicks.
7. In a skillet, heat oil on medium-high heat.
8. Add chicken breast rolls and cook for about 2 minutes per side.
9. Arrange the chicken breast on prepared baking sheet in a single layer.
10. Bake for about 15–20 minutes or until desired doneness.
11. Remove from oven and set aside for about 5 minutes.
12. With a sharp knife, cut into slices and serve.

Nutritional Information (Per Serving)
Calories: 223

Fat: 11.5 g
Sat Fat: 3.7 g
Carbohydrates: 3 g
Fiber: 0.8 g
Sugar: 0.4 g
Protein: 27.3 g
Sodium: 278 mg

Snacks

Tuna on Cukes

Yield: 2 servings
Ingredients:
1 can tuna packed in water
1 cucumber
1 tablespoon mayonnaise
½ stalk celery, chopped
2 tablespoons red onion, minced
1 teaspoon dried basil
1 teaspoon dried oregano
¼ cup fresh sprouts
Salt and pepper to taste

Directions:
1. Slice the cucumber into thick rounds and sprinkle with salt and pepper.

2. Combine the tuna, mayonnaise, celery, onion, and herbs. Mix together. Spoon by the tablespoon onto the cucumber pieces and top with fresh sprouts.

3. Add additional salt and pepper if desired.

Nutritional Information (Per Serving)
Calories: 224
Fat: 9.9 g
Sat Fat: 1.9 g
Carbohydrates: 8.8 g
Fiber: 1.4 g
Sugar: 3.5 g
Protein: 24.9 g

Roasted Seeds and Nuts

Yield: 15 servings
Ingredients:
1 cup almonds
1 cup walnuts
1 cup hazelnuts
1 cup peanuts
½ cup pumpkin seeds
¼ cup sunflower seeds
¼ cup pine nuts
2 sprigs of fresh rosemary
6 leaves of fresh sage
1 teaspoon cayenne pepper
1 tablespoon olive oil
Salt and pepper to taste

Directions:
1. Preheat the oven to 400 degrees F.

2. Spread the nuts and seeds evenly on baking sheet. Sprinkle with cayenne pepper, olive oil, salt, and pepper. Add rosemary and sage.

3. Roast in the oven for about 20 minutes. Remove and allow to cool.

Nutritional Information (Per Serving)
Calories: 228
Fat: 20.9 g
Sat Fat: 2.1 g
Carbohydrates: 6 g
Fiber: 3.1 g
Sugar: 1.1 g
Protein: 8.2 g

Oven Baked Grapefruit

Yield: 2 servings
Ingredients:
1 grapefruit, medium-sized
½ teaspoon ground cinnamon
1 Splenda packet (or comparable sugar substitute)

Directions:
1. Preheat oven to 400 degrees F.
2. Cut grapefruit in half horizontally, using a sharp knife. Using a serrated knife or a grapefruit spoon, loosen segments of fruit, but do not remove from skin.
3. Place halves cut side up on a baking sheet. Sprinkle evenly with cinnamon and sugar substitute. Place in oven and bake for about 20 minutes, or until warmed.
4. Let cool for about 5 minutes before serving. Eat with a grapefruit spoon or serrated spoon or cut up before serving.

Nutritional Information (Per Serving)
Calories: 22
Fat: 0.1 g
Sat Fat: 0 g
Carbohydrates: 5.6 g
Fiber: 1 g
Sugar: 4.5 g
Protein: 0.4 g
Sodium: 0 mg

Edamame and Guacamole

Yield: 6 servings
Ingredients:
2 avocados
1 cup tomatoes, diced
1 clove garlic, minced
¼ cup red onion, diced
8 ounces edamame, steamed
½ lime, juiced
½ teaspoon cayenne pepper
Salt and pepper to taste

Directions:
1. Peel the avocados and remove the pit. Smash it with a fork and stir in the tomatoes, garlic, and red onion.

2. Add the lime juice and cayenne pepper. Sprinkle with salt and pepper.

3. Use the edamame to scoop up the guacamole. Other veggies will work well as dippers too.

Nutritional Information (Per Serving)
Calories: 202
Fat: 15.7 g
Sat Fat: 3.1 g
Carbohydrates: 12.4 g
Fiber: 6.8 g
Sugar: 1.5 g
Protein: 6.6 g

Pumpkin Bars

Yield: 25 servings

Ingredients:

½ cup softened butter

½ cup brown sugar (sugar substitutes are not recommended with this recipe)

½ teaspoon baking soda

½ teaspoon pumpkin pie spice

⅓ cup canned pumpkin

1 egg

1½ cups all-purpose flour

4 ounces cream cheese, softened

1 cup whipped cream

Nutmeg

Directions:

1. Preheat oven to 350 degrees F.

2. Lightly grease and flour a 9x9x2-inch baking dish and set aside.

3. Mix together baking soda, brown sugar, butter, and pumpkin pie spice in a big bowl. Beat the mixture with an electric mixer on medium speed until well-mixed. Add pumpkin and egg. Beat in as much flour as possible. Not all flour will be added in this fashion; the rest must be stirred in using wooden spoon.

4. Spread this dough into the prepared baking dish. Bake for 12 to 15 minutes (until a wooden toothpick can be inserted into the center and come out clean).

5. Let cool for 10 minutes before removing dessert from the dish. Allow to cool.

6. In a medium bowl, use a mixer on medium speed to beat the cream cheese until smooth. Beat in the whipped cream.

7. Spread the mixture over top of the dessert. Sprinkle with nutmeg before cutting into bars.

Nutritional Information (Per Bar)
Calories: 177
Fat: 7.2 g
Sat Fat: 4.4 g
Carbohydrates: 24.4 g
Fiber: 0.8 g
Sugar: 3 g
Protein: 3.6 g
Sodium: 44 mg

Deviled Eggs

Yield: 6 servings
Ingredients:
6 large eggs
1 medium avocado, peeled, pitted, and chopped
2 teaspoons fresh lime juice
Pinch of salt
⅛ teaspoon cayenne pepper

Directions:
1. In a pot of water, hard boil eggs, cooking for about 15–20 minutes.
2. Drain water and let eggs cool completely.
3. Peel eggs and slice in half vertically with sharp knife.
4. Scoop out yolks and transfer half of them to bowl.
5. Add avocado, lime juice, and salt and mash with fork until well combined.
5. Fill egg halves with avocado mixture.
6. Sprinkle with cayenne pepper and serve.

Nutritional Information (Per Serving)
Calories: 140
Fat: 11.5 g
Sat Fat: 2.9 g
Carbohydrates: 3.3 g
Fiber: 2.3 g
Sugar: 0.6 g
Protein: 6.9 g
Sodium: 99 mg

Tomato Bruschetta

Yield: 6 servings

Ingredients:

½ whole-grain baguette, cut into 6 (½-inch-thick) slices on the diagonal

3 tomatoes, chopped

½ cup fennel, chopped

2 garlic cloves, minced

1 tablespoon fresh parsley, chopped

1 tablespoon fresh basil, chopped

2 teaspoons balsamic vinegar

1 teaspoon olive oil

Freshly ground black pepper to taste

Directions:

1. Preheat the oven to broil. Arrange rack in top portion of oven.

2. Arrange bread slices on baking sheet in single layer.

3. Broil for about 2 minutes per side.

4. Meanwhile, in bowl, add remaining ingredients and toss to coat.

5. Divide tomato mixture evenly and place on each slice of toasted bread. Serve immediately.

Nutritional Information (Per Serving)
Calories: 94.5
Fat: 1.5 g
Sat Fat: 0.1 g
Carbohydrates: 18 g
Fiber: 2.5 g
Sugar: 1.0 g
Protein: 3.7 g
Sodium: 176 mg

Dinner

Spicy Chicken Stew

Yield: 6 servings
Ingredients:
2 tablespoons olive oil
1 onion, chopped
½ tablespoon fresh ginger, grated finely
1 tablespoon fresh garlic, minced
1 teaspoon ground coriander
1 teaspoon paprika
1 teaspoon cayenne pepper
6 skinless, boneless chicken thighs, trimmed and cut into 1"
pieces
3 Roma tomatoes, chopped
1 cup coconut milk
1 cup chicken broth
⅓ cup fresh cilantro, chopped
Salt and pepper to taste

Directions:
1. In a large pan, heat oil over medium heat. Add onion and
sauté for 3 minutes.
2. Add ginger, garlic, and spices, and sauté for 1 minute.
3. Add chicken and cook for 4–5 minutes.
4. Add tomatoes, coconut milk, broth, salt, and pepper, and
bring to a gentle simmer.
5. Reduce the heat to low and simmer, covered for about 10–15
minutes or until desired doneness.
6. Stir in cilantro, and remove from heat.

Nutritional Information (Per Serving)
Calories: 167

Fat: 8.8 g
Sat Fat: 2.3 g
Carbohydrates: 7.4 g
Fiber: 1.1 g
Sugar: 4.3 g
Protein: 14.8 g

Meatballs Curry

Yield: 6 servings
Ingredients:
For Meatballs:
1 pound lean ground turkey
2 eggs, beaten
3 tablespoons red onion, minced
¼ cup fresh basil leaves, chopped
¼ teaspoon fresh ginger, chopped finely
4 garlic cloves, chopped finely
1 jalapeño pepper, seeded and minced
1 tablespoon red curry paste
1 tablespoon fish sauce
2 tablespoons coconut oil
Salt to taste

For Curry:
1 red onion, chopped
4 garlic cloves, minced
½ teaspoon fresh ginger, minced
1 jalapeño pepper, seeded and minced
2 tablespoons red curry paste
1 (14 ounces) can coconut milk
2 tablespoons fresh lime juice
Salt and pepper to taste

Directions:

1. For meatballs, in a large bowl, add all ingredients except oil, and mix until well combined. Make small balls from the mixture.

2. In a large skillet, melt coconut oil over medium heat. Add meatballs and cook for 3–5 minutes or until golden brown on all sides. Transfer the meatballs into a bowl.

3. In the same skillet, add onion and a pinch of salt, and sauté for 3 minutes.

4. Add garlic, ginger, and jalapeño, and sauté for 1 minute.

5. Add curry paste, and sauté for 1 minute.

6. Add coconut milk and meatballs, and bring to a gentle simmer. Reduce heat to low and simmer, covered for about 10 minutes.

7. Serve with a drizzling of lime juice.

Nutritional Information (Per Serving)
Calories: 370
Fat: 29.5 g
Sat Fat: 20.8 g
Carbohydrates: 9.8 g
Fiber: 2.2 g
Sugar: 3.7 g
Protein: 19 g

Salmon and Asparagus

Yield: 8 servings

Ingredients:

4 skinless salmon fillets

1 cup sugar snap peas

1 tablespoon fresh chives, snipped

2 leeks, thinly sliced

8 ounces asparagus spears

4 tablespoons dry white wine

1 cup reduced-sodium vegetable broth

Salt and pepper to taste

Directions:

1. Arrange leeks in single layer in a large skillet. Coat with cooking spray. Lay the pieces of salmon on top.

2. Arrange the asparagus and peas around the fish. Sprinkle with wine and broth and season lightly with salt and pepper.

3. Heat the skillet over medium-high heat and wait for the broth to boil. Cover with tight-fitting lid and lower heat.

4. Cook until the salmon is pale pink, even on the inside, and the vegetables are tender. This will take about 12–14 minutes.

5. Once fish is ready, sprinkle with chives and serve.

Nutritional Information (Per Serving)

Calories: 244

Fat: 9.5 g

Sat Fat: 1.4 g

Carbohydrates: 5.3 g

Fiber: 1.2 g

Sugar: 1.8 g

Protein: 30.9 g

Roasted Mackerel

Yield: 4 servings

Ingredients:

8 mackerel fillets

2 garlic cloves, peeled

2 teaspoons paprika

¼ cup green onions, sliced

3 tablespoons olive oil

1 tablespoon white wine vinegar

Salt and pepper to taste

Directions:

1. Preheat oven to 400 degrees F.

2. Press the garlic and paprika together until it becomes a paste. Add some olive oil.

3. Coat the mackerel with olive oil and place on a baking sheet, skin side up. Season with salt and pepper, then cover with the garlic and paprika mixture. Sprinkle the green onions on top.

4. Bake for 10–12 minutes. Remove from the oven and drizzle with vinegar.

5. Serve with your favorite veggie.

Nutritional Information (Per Serving)

Calories: 559

Fat: 42 g

Sat Fat: 8.9 g

Carbohydrates: 1.6 g

Fiber: 0.6 g

Sugar: 0.3 g

Protein: 42.3 g

Cheesy Spinach Bake

Yield: 6 servings
Ingredients:
3 cups spinach
½ cup half & half milk
½ cup milk
3 eggs, beaten
2 egg yolks, beaten
¼ cup butter, melted
1 cup shredded cheddar cheese
2 teaspoons bread crumbs
⅛ teaspoon black pepper
Cooking spray

Directions:
1. Preheat the oven to 350 degrees F. Coat a 2-quart baking dish with cooking spray.

2. Thoroughly clean and dry the spinach before chopping it.

3. Combine cream and milk together in a medium saucepan and heat until near simmering.

4. Combine beaten eggs and yolks together in a medium bowl. Slowly add hot milk and cream, whisking continually until everything is blended together.

5. Add the melted butter slowly while constantly whisking. Add ¾ cup of shredded cheese. Fold the spinach into the dairy and cheese mixture, making sure it is well-combined.

6. Mix remaining cheese and the bread crumbs in a separate bowl. Set the mixture aside.

7. Transfer the spinach mixture into the prepared baking dish. Sprinkle the bread crumb and cheese mixture evenly over top. Bake for 30 minutes.

Nutritional Information (Per Serving)

Calories: 236
Fat: 20.4 g
Sat Fat: 11.8 g
Carbohydrates: 3.6 g
Fiber: 0.4 g
Sugar: 1.4 g
Protein: 10.2 g
Sodium: 240 mg

Vegetarian Chili

Yield: 8 servings
Ingredients:
2 cups onion, diced
1 cup celery, diced
1 cup bell pepper, diced
2 cloves garlic, minced
2 tablespoons water
2 jalapeño peppers, diced
4 cups crushed tomatoes, no salt added
2 cups canned pinto beans, drained and rinsed, no salt added
2 tablespoons cumin
1 tablespoon chipotle pepper
1 tablespoon black pepper
1 tablespoon balsamic vinegar
1 tablespoon oregano

Directions:
1. Add onion, celery, bell pepper, and garlic in 2 tablespoons of water in a stockpot over low heat. Cook until onions are translucent.

2. Add the rest of the ingredients. Cover and simmer for 1–2 hours, occasionally stirring.

3. If chili becomes too thick, thin it with water, adding small increments of water at a time.

Nutritional Information (Per Serving)
Calories: 115
Fat: 1.2 g
Sat Fat: 0.2 g
Carbohydrates: 22.9 g
Fiber: 6.7 g
Sugar: 0.8 g
Protein: 5.6 g
Sodium: 27.1 mg

Ginger Steak

Yield: 4 servings

Ingredients:

8 garlic cloves, crushed

2 teaspoons fresh ginger, sliced thinly

1 tablespoon honey

¼ cup olive oil

Salt and freshly ground black pepper to taste

1½ pounds flank steak, trimmed

Directions:

1. In a large sealable bag, mix together all ingredients except steak.

2. Add steak and coat generously with marinade.

3. Seal the bag, and refrigerate to marinate for about 24 hours.

4. Remove the steak from refrigerator, and keep at room temperature for about 15 minutes.

5. Heat a lightly greased grill pan over medium-high heat. Discard the excess marinade from steak, and place the steak in the grill pan.

7. Cook for 6–8 minutes on each side or until desired doneness.

8. Remove from grill pan, and cool for 10 minutes before slicing.

9. With a sharp knife, cut into desired slices and serve.

Nutritional Information (Per Serving)

Calories: 407

Fat: 26.2 g

Sat Fat: 7.3 g

Carbohydrates: 6.5 g

Fiber: 0.2 g

Sugar: 4.4 g

Protein: 35 g

CHAPTER SIX

Supplement Your Diet

As much as a healthy diet is important for managing type 2 diabetes, you cannot rely solely on balanced meals. When you have diabetes, high blood sugar acts as a diuretic and the nutrients your body absorbed will be filtered out of your body. This makes diabetics prone to deficiency in water-soluble vitamins and minerals. To have a proper nutrition that will keep your blood sugar in check, you need to take supplements. Another reason to take supplements is that by increasing your nutrient intake, you are helping your body use insulin more efficiently to keep your blood glucose levels healthy.

A number of dietary supplements are available for diabetics. Although research on the effectiveness of diabetes supplements is still limited, there are a few supplements that are beneficial. When combined with diabetes diet, regular exercise, and medications, dietary supplements can help manage diabetes and its complications. Make sure to consult your doctor to see which supplement is the best for you. Herbs, for example, can have powerful effects and may interfere with your diabetes medications.

Chromium

Chromium is a trace mineral that can be found in common foods including fruits, vegetables, fish, and meat. Chromium enhances the function of insulin and assists with reducing blood sugar levels. Clinical trials have shown that chromium helps the body distribute glucose and nutrients into cells. However, this supplement should be taken in small doses, as too much chromium can threaten kidney function.

Vitamin D

Diabetics are more prone to infection. Vitamin D activates the immune system and can help you fight bacteria and viruses.

Magnesium

This mineral is essential for protein synthesis and energy production. Studies have shown that increased magnesium intake can slow the progression from pre-diabetes to diabetes.

Prickly Pear Cactus

Some studies have shown that prickly pear cactus lowers blood sugar. Packed with compounds that work much like the insulin, the ripe fruit of this type of cactus can be found in supermarkets or health food stores. Eat it cooked or buy a powdered juice.

Bitter Melon

Do not get confused by its name. Bitter melon is a popular Asian vegetable that is traditionally used as herbal medicine. Bitter melon contains polypeptide-p that acts like insulin to lower blood sugar. Also, bitter melon contains charatin, which promotes the conversion of glucose to glycogen for storage. Although there is limited evidence of clinical studies, bitter melon has shown promise in animal studies as a diabetes supplement. A small amount of its juice daily can have a great impact on your blood sugar.

Aloe Vera

We commonly see aloe vera in many cosmetics products; it has yet another beneficial use. There are studies that have found out that the juice of this plant helps people with type 2 diabetes to lower their blood glucose. Did you know that in Arabia the powdered juice of aloe vera is traditionally used to treat diabetes?

Gymnema Sylvestre Extract

This extract is derived from the leaves of the plant Gymnema sylvestre that grows in the Indian forests. The Gymnemic acids in the extract lower blood glucose by blocking the absorption of sugar. There are limited studies that also show that Gymnema sylvestre extract can regenerate the beta cells in the pancreas that secrete insulin.

Curcumin

Turmeric is a spice that gives curry powder its bright yellow color. Turmeric contains the curcumin compound, which is responsible for the vast majority of the health benefits associated with the spice. Curcumin has also been shown to activate peroxisome proliferator receptors, which are a group of proteins that modulate sugar uptake. In diabetic rats, curcumin has also been shown to improve liver function and lower blood glucose levels. A 9-month research performed on 240 people with pre-diabetes, has shown that those individuals who consume curcumin can prevent diabetes completely.

Cinnamon

Those of you who love cinnamon rolls will definitely love this – studies suggest that consuming a half a teaspoon of cinnamon daily can reduce blood glucose levels and cholesterol.

Fenugreek

A study performed on 25 people has found out that fenugreek has a significant impact on managing blood sugar. Used in the Middle Eastern medicine for over 2000 years, this beneficial spice can help you manage diabetes.

Some of these herbal supplements may interfere with certain medications. Check with your doctor before making these supplements a part of your diet.

Conclusion

If you have type 2 diabetes, managing blood glucose levels should be your top priority. This book cover the most important aspects of a lifestyle that can help you manage blood sugar and beat diabetes.

It's not an easy task to unlearn the unhealthy habits we've accumulated over the years. It's a challenge to change your food preference and to stop yourself from drinking alcohol or smoking. It's hard to start exercising when you just want to stay on the couch and watch TV. However, when you think about the benefits that these lifestyle changes will bring to your health and your life, you'll have the motivation to change for the better.

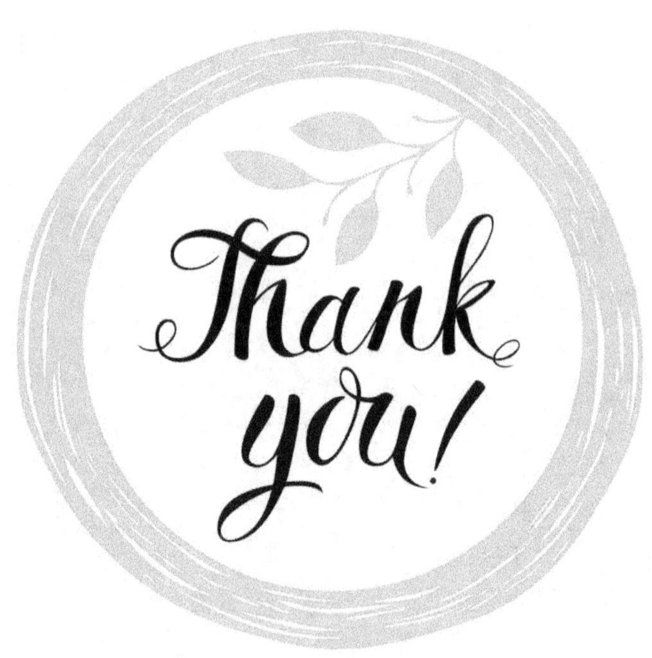

Finally, I want to thank you for reading my book. If you enjoyed the book, please share your thoughts and post a review on the book retailer's website. It would be greatly appreciated!

Best wishes,

Christina Neal